Marma Therapy

A Beginner's 5-Step Quick Start Guide

mf

copyright © 2023 Patrick Marshwell

All rights reserved No part of this book may be reproduced, or stored in a retrieval system, or transmitted in any form or by any means, electronic, mechanical, photocopying, recording, or otherwise, without express written permission of the publisher.

Disclaimer

By reading this disclaimer, you are accepting the terms of the disclaimer in full. If you disagree with this disclaimer, please do not read the guide.

All of the content within this guide is provided for informational and educational purposes only, and should not be accepted as independent medical or other professional advice. The author is not a doctor, physician, nurse, mental health provider, or registered nutritionist/dietician. Therefore, using and reading this guide does not establish any form of a physician-patient relationship.

Always consult with a physician or another qualified health provider with any issues or questions you might have regarding any sort of medical condition. Do not ever disregard any qualified professional medical advice or delay seeking that advice because of anything you have read in this guide. The information in this guide is not intended to be any sort of medical advice and should not be used in lieu of any medical advice by a licensed and qualified medical professional.

The information in this guide has been compiled from a variety of known sources. However, the author cannot attest to or guarantee the accuracy of each source and thus should not be held liable for any errors or omissions.

You acknowledge that the publisher of this guide will not be held liable for any loss or damage of any kind incurred as a result of this guide or the reliance on any information provided within this guide. You acknowledge and agree that you assume all risk and responsibility for any action you undertake in response to the information in this guide.

Using this guide does not guarantee any particular result (e.g., weight loss or a cure). By reading this guide, you acknowledge that there are no guarantees to any specific outcome or results you can expect.

All product names, diet plans, or names used in this guide are for identification purposes only and are the property of their respective owners. The use of these names does not imply endorsement. All other trademarks cited herein are the property of their respective owners.

Where applicable, this guide is not intended to be a substitute for the original work of this diet plan and is, at most, a supplement to the original work for this diet plan and never a direct substitute. This guide is a personal expression of the facts of that diet plan.

Where applicable, persons shown in the cover images are stock photography models and the publisher has obtained the rights to use the images through license agreements with third-party stock image companies.

Table of Contents

Introduction	6
What Is Marma Therapy?	9
Location of Marma Points	10
Benefits of Practicing Marma Therapy	15
Disadvantages of Marma Therapy	20
When You Should Get into Marma Therapy	23
Persistent pain	23
Insomnia	24
Stress	24
Digestive disorders	25
Low energy levels or fatigue	25
Skin conditions	25
Respiratory disorders	26
Heart conditions	26
Difficulty concentrating and/or poor memory	27
How Does Marma Therapy Work?	28
What Should You Expect from a Marma Therapy Session?	34
5-Step Guide on Getting Started the Marma Therapy	35
What You Should Do After Getting Marma Therapy	38
Things You Shouldn't Do After Getting Marma Therapy	42
Foods that Support Marma Therapy	46
Conclusion	49
References and Helpful Links	52

Introduction

If you're looking for a holistic approach to health and well-being, Marma therapy might just be the ticket. This ancient Ayurvedic practice has been around for thousands of years and is all about stimulating specific points in the body to promote healing, relaxation, and rejuvenation.

But don't let the word "ancient" fool you – Marma therapy is backed by science and has been shown to have numerous benefits for physical, emotional, and spiritual well-being. By activating these energy centers throughout the body, you can release blocked energy, improve circulation, and address a wide range of conditions.

So, what exactly is Marma therapy? It's a non-invasive practice that uses gentle pressure, massage, and essential oils to activate Marma points – areas where muscles, veins, arteries, tendons, bones, and joints meet. These points are highly sensitive to touch and manipulation and are said to be gateways to your inner self.

But don't just take our word for it. Studies have shown that Marma therapy can be effective in addressing a range of conditions, including chronic pain, stress, anxiety, and even digestive issues. It can also promote better sleep, boost immunity, and improve overall quality of life.

What's more, Marma therapy is safe and suitable for people of all ages and body types. It's a natural, non-invasive way to promote healing and well-being that doesn't require any expensive equipment or pharmaceutical drugs.

Of course, like any form of therapy, Marma therapy requires commitment and consistency to see lasting results. It's not a one-time fix-it-all solution. But with regular practice, you'll start to notice a profound shift in your overall well-being.

Intrigued? Want to learn more about this ancient practice that's making a comeback? Keep reading! We'll dive deeper into the world of Marma therapy and explore some of its many benefits. So sit back, relax, and get ready to discover the healing power of Marma therapy.

In this guide, we will talk about the following in full detail:

- What is marma therapy?
- Location of Marma Points
- How does it work?
- What are some of the benefits and Some Disadvantages of practicing marma therapy?
- What should you expect from a Marma therapy session?
- How do you get started with marma therapy?

- What You Should and Shouldn't Do After Getting Marma Therapy

By the end of this guide, you'll better understand marma therapy and its many benefits, as well as the necessary steps to get started with your marma therapy practice. Let's dive in!

What Is Marma Therapy?

Marma therapy is an ancient healing practice that has been used in India for over 5,000 years. It's a form of Ayurvedic medicine that focuses on stimulating the body's vital energy points, known as marmas. These energy points are believed to be where the human body's physical, mental, and spiritual aspects converge.

In Sanskrit, the word "marma" means secret or hidden, and marma therapy is all about uncovering these hidden energy points to promote balance and healing throughout the body. Similar to acupressure points in traditional Chinese medicine, marma points are located all over the body, and when stimulated, they can help to release blocked energy, reduce stress, improve circulation, and boost overall health and well-being.

Marma therapy is typically administered through touch, with a practitioner using their hands or fingers to apply pressure to specific points on the body. This pressure can be gentle or firm, depending on the individual's needs and preferences.

Some practitioners may also use essential oils or other natural remedies as part of the treatment.

Location of Marma Points

Marma therapy involves the stimulation of specific points on the body, known as marma points. Here are some of the main marma points and their corresponding locations:

Forehead

Located in the center of the forehead, the marma point associated with the third eye chakra is an important energy center in Ayurvedic medicine. This marma point is believed to enhance intuition and spiritual awareness. It is believed that by activating this marma point, one can improve their spiritual vision, mental clarity, and focus.

It is also believed that this marma point can help with headaches, tension, and stress. It is recommended to massage this marma point with a few drops of warm oil daily to promote overall wellness. Additionally, meditation and yoga practices can help one connect with their third eye chakra and enhance their intuition and spiritual awareness.

Eyebrow Center

The eyebrow center is a vital marma point located between the eyebrows, and it is commonly associated with the pineal gland. This point, when stimulated, can help to improve mental clarity and concentration. The pineal gland is responsible for regulating circadian rhythms and melatonin production, which in turn, affects sleep patterns and mood.

Therefore, when this marma point is activated, it can also lead to a better quality of sleep and enhanced emotional well-being. Given its significance, many traditional healing practices incorporate the use of this point to improve cognitive function and emotional stability. Consequently, by massaging this marma point, one can reap the benefits of heightened mental clarity, concentration, and emotional well-being.

Heart

The Heart marma point is situated in the middle of the chest and is associated with the heart chakra that governs emotions. This vital point is believed to be closely related to emotional equilibrium and promotes overall well-being. It is said that by stimulating this point, one can attain emotional stability, feel empowered and reduce anxiety levels.

This marma point is used in various healing techniques, including Ayurveda and Acupuncture, to boost the immune system and strengthen the heart muscles. Additionally, it is believed to help improve circulation, reduce inflammation, and relieve respiratory issues. Therefore, activating this marma point helps in promoting physical and emotional health.

Navel

The navel, situated in the center of the abdomen, is considered a marma point associated with the solar plexus chakra. It is believed to boost digestive health and vitality. This acupressure point can stimulate the digestive system and help regulate bowel movement.

The manipulation of this point is believed to relieve bloating, constipation, and other digestive issues. Navel stimulation is also thought to activate the body's immune system, strengthen the core, and release stress and tension. Overall, the navel is an important marma point to improve one's overall well-being and digestive health.

Armpit

The armpit marma point, a vital point located in the armpit, is believed to play a critical role in the lymphatic system's detoxification process. Additionally, it is considered to play a significant role in boosting the body's immunity to fight against various diseases. This marma point's activation may stimulate the flow of lymphatic fluids, which helps in the removal of toxins and the body's metabolic waste products.

Furthermore, it can promote the immune system by increasing the production of white blood cells and enhancing the body's defense mechanisms. Overall, activation of this marma point is considered crucial for maintaining optimal health and well-being of an individual.

Knee

The marma point on the inside of the knee joint is essential in Ayurvedic medicine. This point is believed to help alleviate pain and inflammation associated with joint problems. When this point is stimulated, it may enhance the flow of energy through the body, promote healing and rejuvenation, as well as improve the overall mobility and function of the knee.

Regular stimulation of this point may lead to improved joint health and reduced discomfort, helping individuals maintain an active lifestyle.

Palm Heart

Palm Heart is a crucial marma point positioned at the center of the palm, which is strongly linked with the heart chakra that regulates emotions. It is believed that applying pressure on this point can help alleviate anxiety, stress and promote emotional balance.

Besides, many people believe that stimulating this marma can also aid in managing mood swings and enhancing overall well-being. Furthermore, activating the Palm Heart point can promote circulation, improve blood flow, and bring a sense of relaxation to the body and mind.

Temple

The temple point is a vital marma point located on either side of the forehead, above the ears. It is associated with the temporal lobes of the brain and is believed to play a significant role in regulating headaches and migraines.

Applying gentle circular movements on this marma point can help activate the flow of blood and relieve pressure on the head. Moreover, this point is also connected with the eyes and ears, and the stimulation of this area may aid in calming the mind and improving concentration. It is a sensitive spot on the face and massaging it can effectively boost one's general vitality.

Wrist

The marma point located on the wrist is viewed as an important center for the nervous system. Pressure applied to this point is believed to alleviate stress, anxiety, and tension. The wrist marma point is located near major veins and nerves and is considered a sensitive region.

The application of acupressure on this point is believed to activate the brain's release of endorphins, which are known to reduce stress and induce a sense of relaxation. It is believed to provide relief not only from physical pressure and pain but also from emotional stress.

Additionally, it has been suggested that applying consistent pressure on this marma point may also improve circulation and promote overall well-being. When used in conjunction with alternative therapies, like meditation or yoga, pressure to this marma point may be an effective tool to manage stress, anxiety, and tension.

Foot

The foot marma point is situated on the sole of the feet and is linked to the root chakra. Ayurvedic practitioners believe that applying pressure to this point promotes grounding and stability throughout the body.

This marma point is considered essential in Ayurvedic massage therapy as it stimulates the energy flow and promotes a sense of physical and emotional balance. The foot marma point is said to help individuals connect with the earth and cultivate inner strength. Massaging this area can lead to deep relaxation, relieve stress and anxiety, and boost overall well-being.

Marma therapy is a holistic healing practice that utilizes the stimulation of specific points on the body to promote balance and healing in both the physical and subtle energy bodies. It can be used to treat a wide range of conditions, ranging from physical ailments such as joint pain and digestive issues to emotional disturbances like anxiety and depression.

Benefits of Practicing Marma Therapy

Marma therapy is a traditional Indian healing practice that involves manipulating specific energy points in the body to promote physical, mental, and emotional well-being. This ancient technique has been used for centuries to alleviate pain, reduce stress and anxiety, boost the immune system, and restore balance to the body and mind.

Today, many people are turning to marma therapy as a natural and holistic approach to healthcare, with growing evidence supporting its effectiveness. In this chapter, we'll explore some of the benefits of marma therapy and how it can help you achieve optimal health and wellness.

The following benefits of marma therapy include:

Promotes physical relaxation

Marma therapy can be used to calm the body and mind, allowing for deep relaxation. This type of massage is particularly helpful in managing stress, anxiety, and tension. It helps reduce muscle pain and stiffness while calming the nervous system to promote a state of mental clarity and balance.

Boosts mental clarity and balances emotions

By enhancing the flow of oxygen and blood to the brain, marma therapy is believed to improve mental clarity. Marma Therapy is a technique that involves applying pressure to specific acupressure spots all over the body to remove mental blockages and improve mental clarity. It also helps to lower tension and anxiety, both of which may sometimes get in the way of an individual's ability to think clearly and concentrate.

As a consequence of this, Marma Therapy has the potential to assist patients in enhancing their cognitive capacities, memory retention, and general mental function. Attending Marma Therapy sessions regularly can enable one to keep their mental health and overall wellness in the best possible condition.

In addition, Marma Therapy is an efficient method for re-establishing emotional equilibrium. The ancient Indian medicinal practice of applying pressure to certain energy spots on the body that are associated with feelings does so via a technique known as marma point massage. Marma Therapy is a technique that, by applying pressure to specific spots on the body, can assist patients in overcoming emotional blockages and restoring emotional equilibrium.

Individuals who are dealing with stress, anxiety, or depression may find that this therapy is helpful. Marma Therapy can assist individuals in improving both their mental health and their quality of life as a whole by emphasizing the importance of maintaining emotional equilibrium. Therefore, maintaining emotional steadiness and resiliency through regular sessions of Marma Therapy can be beneficial to individuals.

Enhances immune function

By energizing the flow of energy throughout the body, marma therapy is renowned for its capacity to improve immunological function. This therapy can help improve the immune system by applying light and targeted pressure on specific marma points. This is especially good for individuals who are prone to infections or have weaker immunity.

Marma treatment has the potential to be an excellent preventative strategy and a natural way to keep the body healthy and performing at its absolute best. It does this by enhancing overall wellness. It has also been demonstrated through research that marma treatment can assist in the regulation of the body's stress response, which can further contribute to the overall immunological function.

Improves digestion

Marma therapy, a traditional Indian healing technique, can effectively address digestive problems. By applying pressure on certain points in the body, Marma therapy can optimize the functioning of the digestive organs and help eliminate waste products. It is particularly beneficial for those who suffer from bloating, constipation, and other digestive issues.

Marma therapy can stimulate the digestive system, ensuring better nutrient absorption which can help individuals avoid common digestive problems while enhancing overall health. With its numerous benefits, Marma therapy is a highly recommended natural approach to address digestive concerns.

Increases circulation

Marma therapy is an extremely efficient way for enhancing circulation in patients who suffer from insufficient blood flow and edema as a result of their conditions. This helps to promote healthy blood flow throughout the body by eliminating blockages in the energy flow, which in turn helps to improve circulation.

This not only boosts the amount of oxygen and nutrients that are delivered to the cells, but it also lowers the risk of developing circulatory system-related conditions like high blood pressure, coronary artery disease, and varicose veins.

In addition to this, Marma therapy works by stimulating the lymphatic system, which further improves the body's ability to cleanse itself and heal. Marma treatment is a technique that aims to improve one's circulation and promote one's general health and wellness. This approach is natural and holistic.

Overall, marma therapy is a safe and natural way to address physical, mental, emotional, and spiritual imbalances in the body. By stimulating specific energy points in the body, marma therapy can help bring balance and harmony to your well-being. So if you're looking for an alternative approach to healthcare that can provide relief from pain.

Disadvantages of Marma Therapy

Marma therapy is an ancient Indian practice that involves the manipulation of specific points in the body to promote healing and well-being. While this therapy has many benefits, there are also potential disadvantages that should be considered. It's important to be aware of these risks so that you can make an informed decision about whether or not marma therapy is right for you.

In this section, we'll explore some of the potential disadvantages of marma therapy and how they compare to the many benefits of this ancient healing practice. By understanding both the pros and cons of marma therapy, you can make an informed decision about whether or not this treatment is right for your individual needs.

Possible discomfort during therapy

It is crucial to be aware that discomfort or pain may be experienced owing to the application of pressure on specific places of the body when having marma therapy. This is something that should be kept in mind. Even while this discomfort is likely to be fleeting and shouldn't linger for very long, it may nevertheless be cause for anxiety for certain people, even though it is normally brief.

Patients must convey to their therapists any discomfort they may be feeling during treatment so that the level of pressure can be modified appropriately. It is also important to remember that not everyone will suffer discomfort during marma therapy, and the advantages of this ancient Indian healing practice typically surpass any momentary discomfort that may be experienced during treatment.

Risk of injury

A marma therapy session that is carried out incorrectly has the potential to cause severe harm. These injuries are possible outcomes if the treating practitioner lacks the necessary qualifications or experience. Since the treatment entails applying pressure to critical areas of the body, an erroneous application has the potential to cause damage to nerves or tissues, fractures, and even paralysis.

It is essential to select a trained practitioner to gusto the safety and efficacy of the treatment. Patients need to be on the lookout for unqualified practitioners who may put their health in jeopardy by inappropriately administering the treatment.

May not be suitable for everyone

Marma therapy, although beneficial for many individuals, can pose a risk to some people. It's important to consider that marma therapy may not be suitable for those with certain medical conditions or injuries that may be aggravated by the therapy. For example, individuals with cardiovascular disease, high blood pressure, or certain types of cancer should avoid this therapy.

Additionally, pregnant women should avoid marma therapy, as it may stimulate contractions. It's essential to consult with a qualified practitioner before undergoing this therapy to ensure that it's safe and appropriate for individual needs, as adverse effects can occur if not done correctly.

Despite these potential disadvantages, the benefits of marma therapy often outweigh any risks or discomfort associated with the treatment. Marma therapy can help to relieve pain, promote relaxation, reduce stress and anxiety, and improve overall well-being.

It can also help to boost the immune system, improve circulation, and aid in the detoxification process. With proper care and guidance from a qualified practitioner, marma therapy can be a safe and effective treatment option for many people.

When You Should Get into Marma Therapy

When deciding whether or not marma therapy is right for you, it's important to have a thorough understanding of the potential risks and benefits associated with this ancient healing practice. It may be helpful to spend some time exploring different types of therapies and learning more about marma therapy before making a decision.

If you decide that marma therapy is right for you, it's important to select a qualified practitioner that has experience with this type of treatment. It may be helpful to seek recommendations from friends or family members who have used marma therapy in the past or do some research online to find a qualified practitioner.

Here are some of the conditions that may be alleviated with marma therapy:

Persistent pain

Marma therapy has been used since ancient times to alleviate pain and discomfort caused by various conditions. Studies have shown that marma therapy may be beneficial for those suffering from chronic pain, such as arthritis. By applying pressure to specific points on the body known as marmas, it can help to reduce inflammation, improve circulation, and increase the range of motion. Additionally, marma therapy can help to relax muscles and improve flexibility, reducing muscle spasms or other forms of discomfort associated with chronic pain.

Insomnia

Insomnia can create a number of problems, including fatigue, decreased productivity, and poor concentration. Fortunately, marma therapy has the potential to reduce symptoms associated with insomnia. By stimulating the pressure points on the body known as marmas, it can help to relax the nervous system and induce restful sleep. Additionally, marma therapy can help to balance hormones, reduce stress and anxiety, and promote a sense of calmness.

Stress

Stress can have a significant impact on our mental and physical health, leading to feelings of confusion, anxiety, and irritability. Fortunately, marma therapy has the potential to reduce stress levels and improve overall well-being. Stimulating specific points on the body known as marmas, can help to balance hormones, reduce tension in the muscles, and promote relaxation. Additionally, marma therapy can help to boost mood by releasing endorphins, which are hormones that create feelings of joy and happiness.

Digestive disorders

Marma therapy has been shown to improve digestion, reducing symptoms of constipation, indigestion, and other digestive issues. By stimulating certain points on the body known as marmas, marma therapy can increase the flow of digestive juices and help to relax the muscles in the abdominal area. This can reduce bloating, cramping, and gas, while also improving the absorption of nutrients.

Low energy levels or fatigue

Marma therapy can be an effective treatment for fatigue caused by low energy levels. By stimulating specific pressure points on the body, marma therapy helps to balance hormones and increase circulation, resulting in improved energy levels and overall well-being. Additionally, marma therapy can help to reduce stress, boost mood, and promote relaxation, all of which can contribute to increased energy levels and improved overall health.

Skin conditions

Skin diseases like eczema and psoriasis have been proven to be alleviated by marma therapy. It is possible to clear up the skin, reduce inflammation and redness, and enhance circulation by applying pressure to certain spots on the body known as marmas. Marma therapy can also assist to regulate hormones in the body, which can reduce the frequency of flare-ups caused by autoimmune conditions. It is possible to find relief from the skin disorders linked with eczema and psoriasis through the utilization of a treatment plan that involves regular sessions.

Respiratory disorders

On asthma and bronchitis, two of the most common respiratory disorders, marma therapy has been proven to have favorable effects. The pressure that is applied during a marma massage can help to relieve symptoms such as coughing and shortness of breath by reducing inflammation, improving circulation, and relaxing the muscles that surround the lungs. In addition, marma therapy may be helpful in reducing stress and anxiety, both of which may play a role in the exacerbation of respiratory conditions such as asthma and bronchitis.

Heart conditions

For patients suffering from heart issues including high blood pressure, marma therapy has shown to be helpful. Stimulating certain places on the body known as marmas can assist to relax the muscles around the heart and reduce inflammation in the surrounding area. In addition, marma therapy can enhance circulation and lower levels of tension, both of which have a beneficial impact on one's blood pressure levels.

Difficulty concentrating and/or poor memory

Marma therapy can be beneficial for those struggling with difficulty concentrating and poor memory. By stimulating specific points on the body, marma therapy can help to improve focus and alertness, as well as increase blood flow to the brain. This improved circulation can result in increased energy levels and enhanced cognitive performance. Additionally, marma therapy has been found to reduce stress and anxiety, both of which can interfere with concentration and memory.

It is recommended to thoroughly discuss your medical history and any concerns you may have prior to beginning marma therapy. This will help your practitioner determine if marma therapy is appropriate for your needs and can help them create a personalized treatment plan that will provide the most benefit.

Finally, it's important to remember that different people may experience unique benefits from marma therapy. The healing effects of this practice could typically take several sessions before any improvements are noticeable. Results may vary from person to person, and it is important to be patient while waiting for the full effects of marma therapy to take place.

How Does Marma Therapy Work?

Marma therapy works by applying light pressure on specific energy points in the body to help stimulate healing and balance the energy flow. These points, known as marma points, can be found throughout the body and are believed to correspond with certain organs and bodily functions.

When these marma points are stimulated, it can help release blockages in the energy flow, which can lead to improved physical and emotional well-being. Marma therapy is typically performed by an experienced practitioner who will use their hands, fingers, elbows, or other tools to apply pressure on the marma points.

Different Techniques Used In Marma Therapy

Marma therapy can be performed with a variety of different techniques. The practitioner will typically begin with an assessment to determine which marma points need to be addressed and then use one or more techniques to stimulate the desired areas. Some of the most common marma therapy techniques include:

Pressure point application

The technique most utilized in marma therapy is pressure point application. It involves the gentle application of pressure on specific points of the body, which are believed to correspond to various organs, systems, and emotions. These pressure points are located all over the body and are said to be the pathway to the flow of energy or prana.

By manipulating these pressure points, practitioners aim to create balance and harmony in the body's energy system, which enhances overall health and well-being. The effectiveness of this technique has been studied and demonstrated to reduce stress levels, alleviate pain, improve circulation, and promote relaxation.

Massage

Marma therapy massage is a technique that's known for its effectiveness in achieving relaxation. By applying gentle strokes and kneading techniques on the body's soft tissues and muscles, tension is released and circulation is improved. Furthermore, it can help one feel more rejuvenated and energized, as it activates the body's natural healing mechanisms.

This technique has been practiced for thousands of years and has been known to support overall well-being by stimulating specific pressure points in the body. It can also be used to support emotional and psychological health by reducing stress and anxiety levels. Overall, marma therapy massage offers a holistic approach to wellness by addressing both physical and mental health.

Aromatherapy

Aromatherapy is a holistic therapy that uses essential oils to promote relaxation, reduce stress, and improve overall health. By inhaling or applying these natural remedies to the skin, it can help stimulate certain marma points which can play an important role in improving physical and emotional wellbeing. Essential oils have also been known to boost immunity and energy levels, relieve pain and tension, and promote relaxation.

When used in conjunction with other marma therapy techniques, aromatherapy can offer a powerful healing experience that helps to address specific health concerns as well as restore balance to the body's energy system.

Herbal remedies

During marma therapy, herbal medicines are an essential component in providing support for the body's natural healing process. These treatments have been meticulously honed to perfection to cater to the precise requirements and goals of each patient. In some instances, the treatments must be consumed orally, while in others, they must be applied topically to the affected area.

Marma therapy is a technique that involves stimulating certain areas all over the body to assist the body in reaching its full potential in terms of health. Marma therapy is an old technique that can provide the patient with an integrated and all-encompassing method of healing. The patient can increase the therapeutic effect of this technique by using herbal medicines during marma treatment.

Meditation

Marma therapy incorporates meditation as one of its approaches to bring about physical relaxation and harmony throughout the body. Meditation is a practice that involves remaining still and concentrating on one's breathing, or a specific sound or phrase, to bring about mental calmness and a reduction in feelings of tension and worry. Individuals can experience higher well-being, improved mental clarity, and a heightened sense of awareness when meditation is incorporated into the Marma therapy that they are receiving.

In addition, consistent meditation practice can lead to improvements in sleep quality as well as a reduction in the symptoms of both depression and chronic pain. In general, the practice of meditation is a useful tool for enhancing the effects of Marma treatment and fostering optimum health and energy.

Sound therapy

Sound therapy is a powerful technique used in marma therapy to promote relaxation and boost the healing process. Specific sounds or vibrations are used to stimulate the body's natural healing abilities, inducing a deep state of relaxation and reducing stress.

Practitioners may use instruments such as singing bowls or tuning forks to produce specific frequencies that resonate with different parts of the body, promoting a sense of balance and harmony.

This technique is known to have a positive impact on the nervous system, helping to reduce anxiety and depression, and can be used as a complementary treatment for a wide range of health conditions.

Energy work

Marma therapy involves working with the subtle energy fields of the body, which refers to the chakras and meridians. Practitioners utilize various techniques to balance the energy flow in the body, one of which includes Reiki or other forms of energy work.

This method redirects energy by laying hands on specific acupressure points in the body. Its goal is to release blockages and promote healing, thereby stimulating the body's natural ability to self-heal. Reiki is seen as a powerful and effective approach to addressing physical, emotional, and spiritual imbalances.

Yoga

Marma therapy practitioners often combine the technique with yoga postures or breathing exercises to enhance the benefits of the treatment. These additional techniques can promote flexibility, balance, and strength, which lead to improved physical health and emotional well-being.

By incorporating yoga into marma therapy, practitioners may offer a more comprehensive approach to healing, targeting both the body and mind. In addition, yoga poses and breathing techniques can also alleviate stress and tension in the body, further aiding in the healing process.

Overall, marma therapy is a holistic approach to healing and wellness that incorporates a variety of techniques to promote balance and harmony in the body, mind, and spirit. By working with a qualified practitioner, individuals can experience a wide range of benefits, from physical relaxation to emotional healing and spiritual growth.

What Should You Expect from a Marma Therapy Session?

A Marma therapy session typically lasts anywhere from one to two hours. During this time, the practitioner will assess any areas of concern and design a customized treatment plan based on the individual's needs. The practitioner may use a variety of techniques during the session, including pressure point application, massage, aromatherapy, herbal remedies, meditation, sound therapy, color therapy, energy work, and yoga.

At the end of the session, the practitioner will usually provide advice on how to continue self-care at home. This may include lifestyle changes or recommendations for further treatments or therapies. It is important to follow these instructions to maximize the benefits of your Marma therapy experience.

5-Step Guide on Getting Started the Marma Therapy

Once you've decided to pursue Marma therapy, there are a few steps you can take to ensure a positive experience. Following this 5-step guide will help you get the most out of your Marma therapy sessions.

Here's a 5-step guide on getting started with Marma Therapy:

Step 1: Learn the Basics

To begin with Marma Therapy, one should have a strong foundation of the basics. The history of Marma Therapy is fascinating and can provide insight into how it has evolved. Understanding the principles of Marma Therapy is essential for proper treatment and care.

Each energy center in the body plays a crucial role in balancing and restoring the body's natural energy flow. Therefore, it's vital to have a comprehensive grasp of these concepts before embarking on Marma Therapy. With a solid foundation, one can use Marma Therapy effectively to promote healing, vitality, and overall well-being.

Step 2: Identify Your Marma Points

In the next step, one must first identify their own Marma points. These are crucial points on the body where energy flows, and there are 107 in total, each with a unique function. Understanding these points is the basis of Marma Therapy.

By identifying these points, individuals can work to improve their well-being and overall health. It's important to focus on this step before beginning treatment, as it sets the foundation for the entire process. Taking the time to learn about one's own Marma points is a key step in achieving optimal health and wellness.

Step 3: Understand the Benefits and Risks

It is crucial to thoroughly comprehend the potential benefits and risks involved. The technique may confer benefits such as reduced anxiety, stress, and chronic pain, among others. However, it should be pursued with care, and if there are any doubts or concerns, it is recommended that healthcare professionals are consulted.

Maintaining a healthy skepticism and being alert to any problems that arise during treatment is also important. The patient should prioritize their safety and well-being at all times during the treatment.

Step 4: Choose Your Technique

It is essential to choose the right technique. One must consider their preferences, comfort level, and health condition before selecting a technique that aligns well with them. Massage, acupressure, and pranic healing are some common techniques used in Marma Therapy.

Each technique has its unique benefits and is effective in treating specific health issues. Therefore, one should conduct proper research and seek professional advice before settling on a technique. A well-informed decision will ensure that the individual gets the maximum benefits of Marma therapy.

Step 5: Practice Regularly

It's important to understand the significance of practicing regularly. Consistency in this practice helps ensure that your body's energy levels remain balanced, leading to a more relaxed state of mind. Whether one is looking to manage stress or cope with specific health concerns, regular Marma Therapy sessions can improve overall well-being.

It's recommended to set aside a few hours each week to practice and make it a part of one's daily routine. The more one practices, the more they will reap the benefits of this ancient medicinal practice.

Overall, marma therapy can be a powerful tool for promoting health and wellness, but it's important to approach it with care and caution. By following these steps and working with a qualified practitioner, individuals can experience a wide range of benefits, from improved physical function to emotional healing and spiritual growth.

What You Should Do After Getting Marma Therapy

Once you have experienced the benefits of Marma therapy, it is important to continue taking proactive steps for maintaining your health and well-being. There are a variety of self-care practices that can be incorporated into your everyday life to ensure that you reap all of the ongoing benefits from Marma therapy.

Here are a few tips on how you can best:

Take rest

After receiving Marma's therapy, it's important to prioritize getting adequate rest. This will allow the body to heal and recharge. Aim to get 7-8 hours of sleep each night to prevent burnout and exhaustion. Lack of sleep can lead to a weakened immune system, increased stress levels, and impaired cognitive function.

Additionally, research has shown that sleep deficiency can also increase the risk of developing chronic health conditions, such as obesity and diabetes. Prioritizing rest is therefore essential for maintaining overall health and well-being.

Drink plenty of water

It is highly recommended to drink a considerable amount of water after marma therapy. This is because the therapy facilitates the elimination of toxins from the body. These toxins are often released into the bloodstream and therefore, drinking plenty of water is essential to assist in flushing them out.

Staying adequately hydrated, allows the body to remove toxins more efficiently, which promotes good health and prevents dehydration. It is advisable to drink a minimum of two to three liters of water daily, especially after receiving marma therapy. Doing so will maximize the benefits of the therapy and ensure optimal recovery.

Avoid caffeine, alcohol, and heavy meals

After getting marma therapy, it is crucial to avoid substances that can disrupt the healing process. Caffeine and alcohol can cause dehydration, which can delay the body's recovery. Heavy meals can also slow down the digestive system, making it harder for the body to absorb nutrients.

Therefore, it's recommended to stick to light and healthy foods and drinks, such as fruits, vegetables, and water. These substances can promote healing by supplying the body with essential nutrients and preventing inflammation. By following these simple guidelines, the individual can optimize their healing process and achieve the maximum benefits of marma therapy.

Practice gentle stretching or yoga

Following marma therapy, it's advisable to practice gentle stretching or yoga to further enhance relaxation and promote healing in the body. Such practices can also help improve flexibility, range of motion, and circulation, in addition to reducing stress and anxiety levels.

Whether it's a few basic stretches or a more advanced yoga session, post-marma therapy stretching can help your body release tension, leaving you feeling refreshed and energized. So, don't forget to incorporate some light stretching or yoga post-marma therapy for optimal benefits.

Avoid exposure to extreme weather conditions

After receiving marma therapy, it is recommended that individuals avoid exposure to extreme weather conditions for at least two to three hours. The therapy stimulates the body's natural healing process, which can leave it vulnerable to stressors such as extreme heat or cold.

By avoiding these conditions, the body can recover properly and maintain the benefits of the therapy. Additionally, extreme weather can lead to dehydration and fatigue, negatively impacting the body's ability to heal. It is important to prioritize rest and self-care in the hours following marma therapy for optimal results.

Take a warm bath or shower

After receiving marma therapy, it is highly recommended to take a warm bath or shower to further aid in muscle relaxation and healing. The warmth of the water can help increase blood flow and reduce inflammation, which can promote faster recovery.

Additionally, adding Epsom salts to the bathwater can provide added benefits, such as relieving muscle soreness and tension. Epsom salts contain magnesium, which can help soothe the nervous system and induce relaxation. This simple post-therapy ritual can greatly enhance the overall effectiveness of the marma therapy treatment.

Listen to your body

After getting marma therapy, it is essential to be mindful of your body's response. It is recommended to pay attention to how your body feels and to adjust your activities accordingly. If you feel tired or sore, it is best to take things slow and give yourself the time you need to fully recover.

It is also important to note that this therapy can have varying effects on individuals, with some experiencing immediate relief, while others may need to continue the treatment.

Therefore, it is advisable to consult with your therapist and follow their guidance on how to manage your symptoms after the treatment. Taking care of yourself post-treatment can maximize the benefits of marma therapy and enhance your overall well-being.

By following these tips and working with a qualified practitioner, individuals can experience a wide range of benefits from marma therapy. With the right preparation and follow-up care, individuals can optimize their healing potential and enjoy all of the positive effects of this powerful holistic treatment.

Things You Shouldn't Do After Getting Marma Therapy

It is just as important to know what not to do after getting marma therapy, to ensure that you get the most out of your treatment.

Below are some key activities and behaviors to avoid after receiving marma therapy:

Engage in strenuous physical activities

It is crucial to refrain from any strenuous physical activities after receiving marma therapy. The reason lies in the fact that muscles and joints require sufficient time to recover and heal from the treatment. Engaging in any rigorous activity too soon after therapy would not only negate its benefits but could also lead to injury or strain on the body.

Therefore, it is imperative to avoid activities such as weightlifting, running, or excessive physical exertion for a significant period after the procedure. Giving the body sufficient rest post-therapy can help optimize its effectiveness and lead to better overall outcomes.

Taking a cold shower

After receiving marma therapy, one should avoid taking a cold shower. The sudden shock of cold water can cause the muscles to contract, exacerbating any soreness or pain from the therapy. Instead, a warm shower or bath is recommended to aid in relaxation and promote therapeutic healing.

It is important to note that the effects of marma therapy can differ for everyone, and it is crucial to listen to one's body and avoid activities that may cause discomfort or hinder the healing process. Always consult with a trained practitioner before undergoing any type of therapy.

Engage in stressful activities

After receiving marma therapy, it is important to avoid any activities that may induce stress. This includes anything that requires physical exertion or mental strain. Engaging in stressful activities may cause tension in the muscles, which can hinder the healing process.

Instead, it is recommended to focus on relaxing activities such as meditation, gentle yoga, or stretching. These activities promote relaxation and aid in the healing process. It is also important to hydrate and rest after marma therapy to allow the body to fully recover.

Neglect self-care practices

It is crucial for individuals who have undergone marma therapy to avoid neglecting necessary self-care practices thereafter. Failing to prioritize activities such as drinking ample water, consuming nutritious foods, and acquiring enough quality rest may impede the healing process and prolong recovery time.

These actions are intrinsic to the body's ability to regenerate and attain optimal health. Therefore, it is advisable to adhere to these self-care practices to bolster the effectiveness of marma therapy and facilitate a speedy recovery.

Overdo it with physical therapy or exercise

After receiving marma therapy, it is important to be mindful of physical activity and exercise. To avoid injury and interfere with the healing process, it is advised to avoid overdoing physical therapy or exercise.

This means avoiding high-intensity workouts, heavy lifting, or excessive stretching. It is recommended that patients engage in gentle physical activity and gradually increase intensity over time. Consulting with a healthcare professional or certified fitness instructor can also help determine an appropriate exercise routine after marma therapy.

Ignore any discomfort or pain

After receiving marma therapy, individuals should not disregard any discomfort or pain experienced in the treated area. It is crucial to pay attention to these sensations as disregarding them may result in further injury or delay in the healing process.

It is advised to seek consultation with a healthcare provider if one experiences persistent or severe discomfort or pain. It is important to take precautions and follow post-treatment care instructions to ensure a smooth and successful recovery.

Following these guidelines after receiving marma therapy is essential for optimal recovery and the best possible outcome. By avoiding these activities, one can ensure effective healing and a speedy recovery.

Foods that Support Marma Therapy

In addition to following the tips outlined in the previous chapter, consuming certain foods can also aid in marma therapy. Including specific types of food and herbs in one's diet may optimize its benefits and further promote relaxation.

Here's a list of foods that can support marma therapy to enhance its effects:

- *Warm soups:* Soups made with nourishing ingredients like vegetables and bone broth can help support digestive health and promote overall well-being.
- *Fresh fruits and vegetables:* Fruits and vegetables are rich in essential vitamins, minerals, and antioxidants that can help boost the immune system and support overall health.
- *Whole grains:* Whole grains like brown rice, quinoa, and oats are a great source of complex carbohydrates and fiber, which can help regulate blood sugar levels and support digestion.

- *Healthy fats:* Healthy fats like avocado, olive oil, and nuts can help support brain function and improve heart health.
- *Herbal teas:* Herbal teas like chamomile, mint, and ginger can help soothe the body and support relaxation.
- *Spices:* Spices like turmeric, cinnamon, and cumin are believed to have anti-inflammatory properties that can help reduce inflammation in the body.
- *Legumes:* Legumes like beans and lentils are a great source of plant-based protein and fiber, which can help support digestive health and regulate blood sugar levels.
- *Healthy beverages:* Beverages like coconut water and green tea can help hydrate the body and provide essential nutrients.
- *Fermented foods:* Fermented foods like kimchi and sauerkraut are rich in beneficial bacteria that can help support gut health and boost the immune system.
- *Dark chocolate:* Dark chocolate is rich in antioxidants and may help improve mood and cognitive function.

Incorporating the right foods into your diet can help enhance the effects of marma therapy and promote overall wellness. By incorporating warm soups, fresh fruits and vegetables, whole grains, healthy fats, herbal teas, spices, legumes, healthy beverages, fermented foods, and dark chocolate, you can provide your body with the essential nutrients it needs to function at its best.

Whether you're new to marma therapy or a seasoned practitioner, these foods can help support your journey towards optimal health and well-being.

Conclusion

Congratulations! You made it to the end of our Marma Therapy journey. We hope that you found this guide informative, inspiring, and maybe even a little bit amusing. Throughout this series, we have explored the ancient Indian healing practice of Marma Therapy, and hopefully, you now have a deeper understanding of its benefits.

Marma Therapy is a holistic system of healing that focuses on balancing the body, mind, and spirit. The techniques used in Marma Therapy are simple, yet powerful, and can be used to address a wide range of physical, emotional, and spiritual issues.

Some of the benefits of Marma Therapy include reducing stress and anxiety, improving digestion, boosting energy levels, and promoting overall well-being.

One of the things that make Marma Therapy so special is that it is a non-invasive, gentle, and holistic approach to healing. Unlike many Western medical treatments, which tend to focus solely on treating symptoms, Marma Therapy aims to address the underlying causes of imbalances in the body. By doing so, it helps to promote long-term healing and well-being.

Another great thing about Marma Therapy is that it is accessible to everyone. You don't need any special equipment or training to start practicing it. All you need is your own two hands and a willingness to learn. Whether you choose to work with a trained Marma Therapy practitioner or practice on your own, the benefits of Marma Therapy are available to you.

If you're new to Marma Therapy, we recommend starting slow and taking the time to learn the basics. There are many resources available online that can help you get started, including videos, articles, and books. You might also consider attending a workshop or class to learn more about Marma Therapy and to connect with others who share your interests.

As you become more familiar with Marma Therapy, you can begin to explore more advanced techniques, such as herbal remedies, meditation, and yoga. These practices can be used in conjunction with Marma Therapy to promote even greater healing and well-being.

One of the most important things to keep in mind when practicing Marma Therapy is that it is a journey, not a destination. Healing takes time, patience, and dedication, but the rewards are well worth the effort. Remember to be gentle with yourself as you learn and grow, and don't be afraid to ask for help or support when you need it.

In conclusion, Marma Therapy is a powerful and transformative practice that can help you achieve greater health and well-being. It offers many benefits, including reduced stress and anxiety, improved digestion, increased energy levels, and a greater sense of overall happiness and contentment. We encourage you to explore this ancient healing art and to see for yourself how it can improve your life. Take the first step today and start your own Marma Therapy journey. You won't regret it.

References and Helpful Links

What Are Marma Points in Ayurveda Healing? (2020, September 30). Healthline. https://www.healthline.com/health/marma

Tnn. (2019, November 12). Marma, the life changing Ayurvedic therapy and the foods which support it. The Times of India. https://timesofindia.indiatimes.com/life-style/food-news/marma-the-life-changing-ayurvedic-therapy-and-the-foods-which-support-it/articleshow/72019647.cms

Fox, M. K., Dickens, A., Greaves, C., Dixon, M. J., & James, M. W. (2006). MARMA THERAPY FOR STROKE REHABILITATION – A PILOT STUDY. Journal of Rehabilitation Medicine, 38(4), 268–271. https://doi.org/10.1080/16501970600630820

Marma Therapy — Moksha Massage. (n.d.). Moksha Massage. https://mokshacolumbus.com/marma-therapy

Gautam, A. K., Verma, P., & Pathak, A. K. (2021). Blood pressure normalizing effect of Talahridaya marma therapy: A case report. Journal of Ayurveda and Integrative Medicine, 12(3), 553–555. https://doi.org/10.1016/j.jaim.2021.05.014

Ayurveda Marma Chikiltsa Ajman | Marma Massage | Marma Therapy. (n.d.). alshifaayurveda.ae.
https://www.alshifaayurveda.ae/therapy/marma-chikiltsa

Marma - Touch Point Therapy — Ayurveda Vancouver. (n.d.). Ayurveda Vancouver.
https://www.ayurvedavancouver.com/treatments/marma-touch-point-therapy

www.ingramcontent.com/pod-product-compliance
Lightning Source LLC
LaVergne TN
LVHW010436070526
838199LV00066B/6048